OSTEOPOROSIS DIET COOKBOOK FOR WOMEN

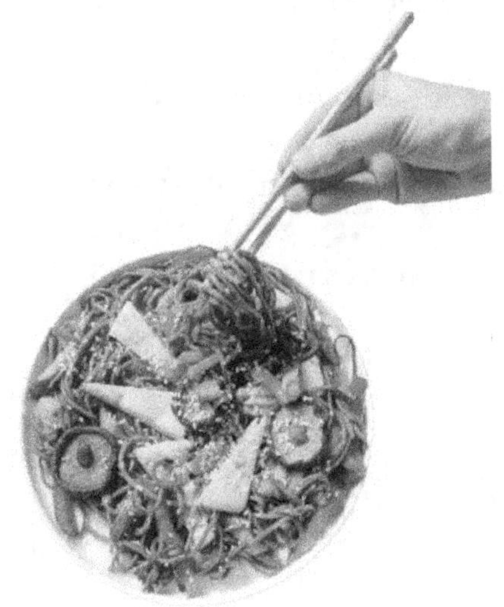

Discover Delicious and Calcium-Rich Recipes with a 30-Day Meal Plan for Optimal Bone Health

ARIA G JAMES

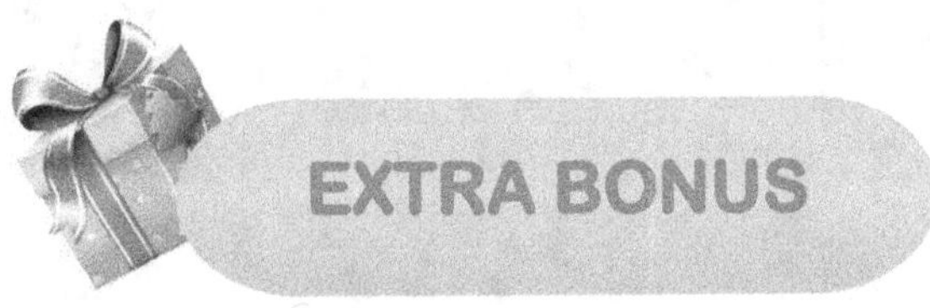

BONUS NO. 1

20-SUITABLE EXERCISES

FOR BONE HEALTH

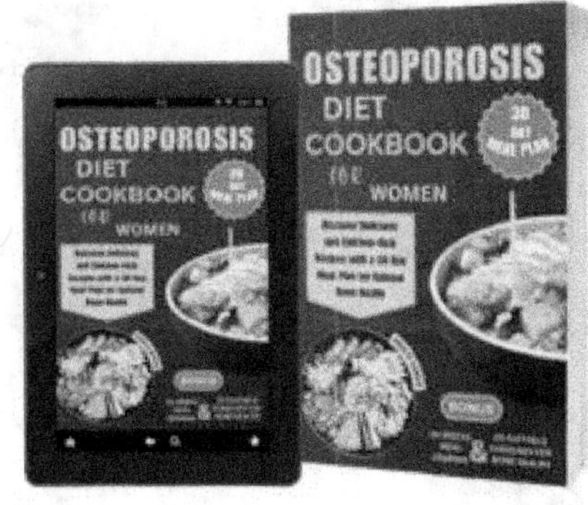

BONUS NO. 2

20-WEEKS MEAL

JOURNAL

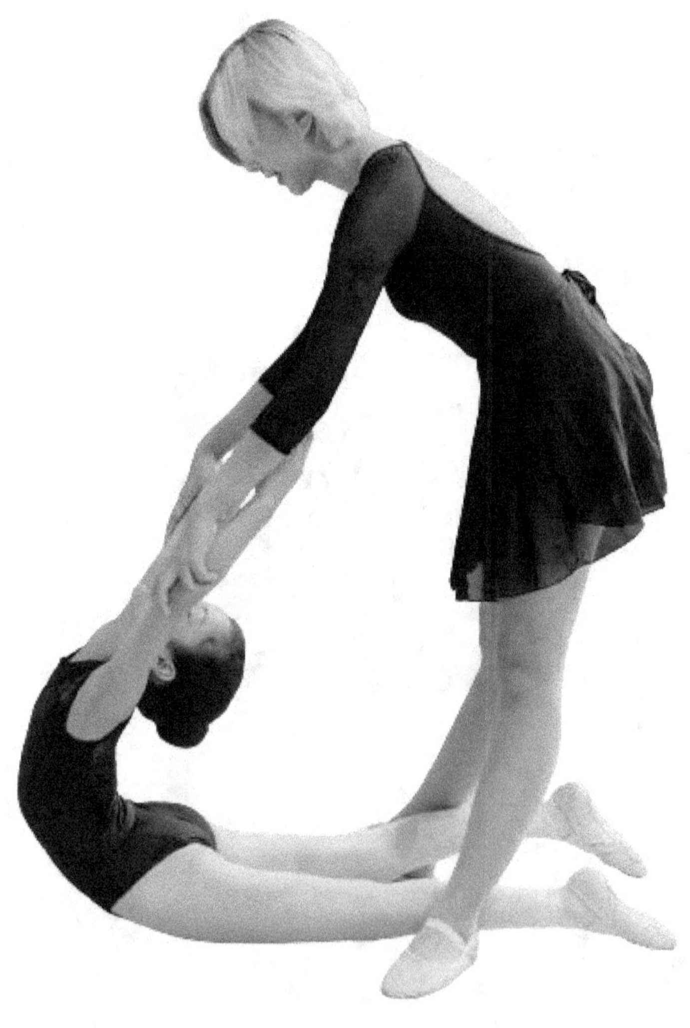

TABLE OF CONTENTS

INTRODUCTION

Welcome to the "Osteoporosis Diet Cookbook for Women." In this comprehensive guide, we embark on a journey to empower women with the knowledge and tools necessary to enhance their bone health through a nourishing and delightful culinary experience.

Osteoporosis, a condition characterized by weakened and brittle bones, is a prevalent concern, especially among women. This cookbook is meticulously crafted to address the intricacies of osteoporosis, offering not only an understanding of its nuances but also practical solutions through the powerful medium of nutrition. By combining the latest insights on osteoporosis with delicious, calcium-rich recipes, we aim to inspire a proactive approach to bone health.

In the initial chapters, we delve into the fundamentals of osteoporosis, unraveling its types, causes, symptoms, and preventive measures. Understanding the risk factors specific to women becomes the cornerstone of our exploration, paving the way for an in-depth examination of the pivotal role nutrition plays in bone health.

The subsequent chapters are dedicated to building a strong foundation for bone health. We navigate through the basics, providing insights into the intricate relationship between diet and bone density. The heart of the book lies in the practical application of this knowledge – a 30-day meal plan meticulously designed to fortify bones, accompanied by a handy grocery shopping guide and quick meal prep tips.

Our journey continues with a detailed exploration of osteoporosis-friendly foods, ensuring that every bite contributes to bone strength. The centerpiece of this culinary odyssey is a collection of delicious and nourishing recipes, thoughtfully categorized into breakfast boosts, lunches for bone support, dinners for building better bones, and snacks and treats that promote healthy bones.

As a bonus, we present a curated list of 20 suitable exercises for bone health, recognizing the holistic approach necessary for optimal well-being. To encourage mindful eating and track progress, a weekly meal journal is also included.

This book is more than a compilation of recipes; it's a guide to a lifestyle that prioritizes bone health without compromising on flavor or variety. We invite you to embark on this culinary and educational adventure, arming yourself with the tools to nurture your bones and embrace a life of strength, vitality, and well-being.

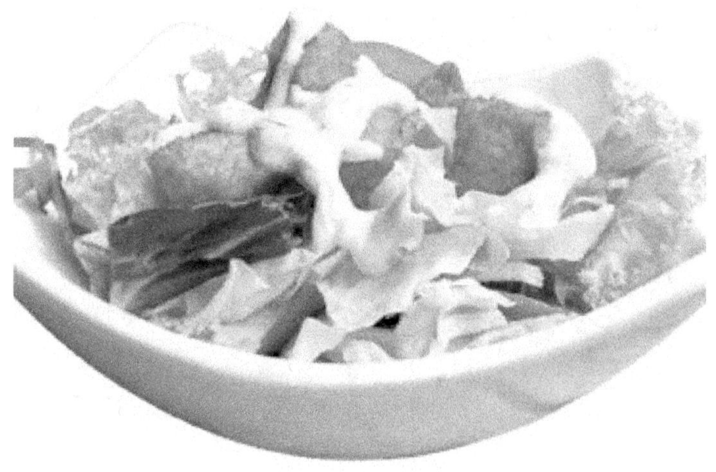

CHAPTER 1

UNDERSTANDING OSTEOPOROSIS

Osteoporosis, a condition often underestimated until its effects become apparent, is a silent but significant threat to bone health. In this section, we delve into the intricacies of osteoporosis, providing a thorough understanding of its nature, types, causes, symptoms, and preventive measures.

What is Osteoporosis?

Osteoporosis is a systemic skeletal disorder characterized by a reduction in bone density and quality. This weakening of bones results in an increased susceptibility to fractures, particularly in weight-bearing bones such as the spine, hips, and wrists. The condition develops slowly over time, often without noticeable symptoms until a fracture occurs. Essentially, osteoporosis compromises the structural integrity of bones, making them more porous and fragile.

Types of Osteoporosis

Understanding the different types of osteoporosis is essential for tailoring preventive measures to individual circumstances.

Postmenopausal Osteoporosis: This type is commonly observed in women after menopause due to a decline in estrogen levels, which plays a crucial role in bone density maintenance.

Senile Osteoporosis: Occurring with aging, senile osteoporosis affects both men and women and is associated with the natural bone loss that comes with aging.

Secondary Osteoporosis: Resulting from underlying medical conditions, medications, or treatments, secondary osteoporosis underscores the importance of addressing root causes for effective management.

Causes of Osteoporosis

Several factors contribute to the development of osteoporosis, creating a complex interplay that impacts bone health.

Hormonal Changes: Postmenopausal women, due to decreased estrogen levels, are particularly susceptible.

Genetic Predisposition: Family history can influence susceptibility to osteoporosis.

Lifestyle Choices: Inadequate calcium and vitamin D intake, sedentary lifestyles, smoking, and excessive alcohol consumption are significant contributors.

Medical Conditions and Medications: Conditions such as rheumatoid arthritis and certain medications like corticosteroids can accelerate bone loss.

Symptoms of Osteoporosis

Osteoporosis is often asymptomatic until fractures occur, but certain signs may indicate its presence:

Back Pain: Especially in the lower back, resulting from fractured or collapsed vertebrae.

Loss of Height: Compression fractures in the spine can lead to a gradual loss of height.

Increased Fracture Risk: Fragile bones increase susceptibility to fractures, even with minor trauma.

Preventive Measures for Osteoporosis

Preventing osteoporosis involves a multifaceted approach:

Dietary Considerations: Ensure an adequate intake of calcium and vitamin D through a balanced diet or supplements.

Regular Exercise: Weight-bearing exercises and resistance training enhance bone density.

Healthy Lifestyle Choices: Quit smoking, limit alcohol intake, and maintain a healthy body weight.

Medical Check-ups: Regular screenings and bone density tests can identify risk factors and enable early intervention.

Medication, if Necessary: In some cases, medications may be prescribed to slow down bone loss.

CHAPTER 2

RISK FACTORS FOR OSTEOPOROSIS IN WOMEN

Osteoporosis, a condition characterized by reduced bone density and increased susceptibility to fractures, is a significant concern, particularly for women. In this comprehensive exploration, we delve into the unique risk factors associated with osteoporosis in women, emphasizing the crucial role of nutrition in maintaining optimal bone health. As we embark on this journey, we aim to provide not just information but a practical guide within the context of our cookbook, "Osteoporosis Diet Cookbook for Women."

Understanding the Risk Factors for Women's Osteoporosis

Osteoporosis affects millions of women globally, and certain risk factors heighten their vulnerability to this condition. One of the primary factors is age, with bone density naturally declining as women age, especially after menopause. Estrogen, a hormone that plays a key role in maintaining bone density, diminishes during menopause, accelerating bone loss.

Genetics also play a crucial role. Women with a family history of osteoporosis are at a higher risk, underscoring the importance of understanding one's genetic predisposition. Additionally, a petite or thin build can increase susceptibility, as there is less bone mass to draw from as women age.

Another important risk factor is a sedentary lifestyle. Weight-bearing exercises stimulate bone formation, and the absence of such activities contributes to reduced bone density. Smoking and excessive alcohol consumption further compound the risk, as these habits have detrimental effects on bone health.

The Importance of Nutrition for Bone Health

The foundation of bone health is laid in the choices we make at the dinner table. Nutrition is not merely a component of overall health; it is a cornerstone in the prevention and management of osteoporosis.

Our bodies continuously undergo bone remodeling, a process where old bone is replaced by new bone tissue. This intricate dance requires an array of nutrients, each playing a unique role.

Calcium, the most abundant mineral in bones, is critical for their strength and structure. Adequate calcium intake is essential, and while dairy products are commonly associated with calcium, leafy green vegetables, fortified plant-based milk, and almonds offer excellent alternatives.

Vitamin D is a key player in calcium absorption, facilitating its incorporation into the bones. Exposure to sunlight is a natural source of vitamin D, but dietary sources such as fatty fish, fortified cereals, and egg yolks are crucial, especially for those with limited sun exposure.

Proteins contribute to bone structure and density, making it imperative to include lean proteins in one's diet. A balance of meats, poultry, fish, beans, and legumes ensures a diverse and nutrient-rich protein intake.

Magnesium, often overlooked, is instrumental in bone mineralization. Nuts, seeds, whole grains, and leafy greens are valuable sources of magnesium that complement calcium and contribute to overall bone health.

Phosphorus, found in various foods including meat, dairy, and nuts, is another essential mineral in bone composition. Striking a balance between phosphorus and calcium intake is crucial for maintaining bone health.

How Diet Affects Bone Density

Dietary choices exert a profound influence on bone density, directly impacting the body's ability to build and maintain strong bones. Adequate calcium intake is non-negotiable, as bones act as a reservoir for calcium. When dietary calcium is insufficient, the body extracts calcium from bones, compromising their density over time.

Conversely, a diet rich in the necessary nutrients promotes bone mineralization. Vitamin D enhances the absorption of calcium, ensuring its effective utilization in bone formation. Proteins provide the necessary amino acids for collagen formation, a structural component of bones. Magnesium and phosphorus work synergistically with calcium, contributing to the intricate matrix that constitutes bone tissue.

Moreover, the balance between acidity and alkalinity in the body, often referred to as the acid-base balance, influences bone health. Diets high in acid-producing foods, such as excessive meat or caffeine, may lead to increased calcium loss through urine. On the other hand, diets rich in fruits and vegetables, despite their natural acidity, have an alkalizing effect, promoting a favorable environment for bone health.

Foods to Include and Foods to Avoid

Navigating the grocery aisles with a keen awareness of bone health transforms the act of shopping into a proactive step toward preventing osteoporosis. Our cookbook provides a curated list of foods that serve as allies in fortifying bones and those that are best approached with caution.

Foods to Include:

Calcium-Rich Sources: Dairy products are well-known sources of calcium, but for those with lactose intolerance or dietary preferences, alternatives like fortified plant-based milk, leafy green vegetables (such as kale and broccoli), and almonds are excellent choices.

Vitamin D Enriched Foods: Fatty fish, such as salmon and mackerel, are not only rich in omega-3 fatty acids but also provide vitamin D. Fortified cereals and egg yolks are additional sources for those seeking dietary alternatives.

Lean Proteins: Incorporating a variety of lean proteins into the diet is vital for bone health. This includes poultry, fish, lean cuts of meat, beans, and legumes.

Magnesium-Loaded Options: Nuts, seeds, whole grains, and leafy greens offer abundant magnesium, supporting the bone mineralization process.

Foods to Approach with Caution:

Excessive Salt Intake: High sodium consumption can lead to calcium loss through urine, potentially weakening bones. A mindful approach to salt intake, including reading food labels and avoiding heavily processed foods, is advised.

Limiting Caffeine and Alcohol: While moderate consumption of caffeine and alcohol may not pose significant risks, excessive intake can interfere with calcium absorption. Balancing these beverages with adequate water intake and calcium-rich foods is recommended.

Phosphoric Acid in Soda: Certain sodas with high phosphoric acid content may interfere with calcium absorption. Limiting the consumption of these beverages contributes to maintaining a healthy acid-base balance.

In the realm of bone health, knowledge is empowerment. Armed with an understanding of the risk factors unique to women, the foundational importance of nutrition, and the intricate ways in which diet affects bone density, women can make informed choices that resonate throughout their lives.

Our cookbook transcends the realm of a mere recipe collection; it becomes a trusted guide for women to nourish their bones with every bite. By incorporating delicious and nutrient-dense recipes, we aim not only to inspire healthier eating but also to infuse joy into the journey toward stronger bones. It's not just about the meals on the table; it's about cultivating a lifestyle that celebrates and sustains the resilience of women's bones.

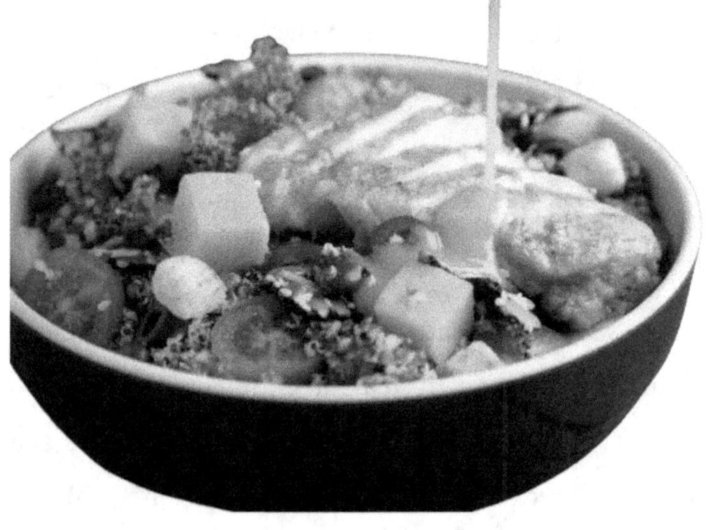

CHAPTER 3

OSTEOPOROSIS-FRIENDLY FOODS

In the pursuit of optimal bone health and the prevention of osteoporosis, the role of nutrition takes center stage. Choosing the right foods can contribute significantly to bone strength, density, and overall well-being. In this chapter we explore a variety of osteoporosis-friendly foods that form the backbone of a diet designed to promote and maintain robust bone health.

1. Dairy Products:

Dairy products are renowned for their high calcium content, a mineral essential for bone strength. Milk, yogurt, and cheese are excellent sources of calcium, and they also provide vitamin D, which is crucial for calcium absorption. For those who are lactose intolerant or choose plant-based alternatives, fortified plant milks, such as almond or soy milk, can be valuable substitutes.

2. Leafy Green Vegetables:

Leafy greens are nutritional powerhouses rich in calcium, magnesium, and vitamin K, all essential for bone health. Incorporate kale, collard greens, spinach, and broccoli into your meals to boost your nutrient intake. These vegetables provide a diverse range of vitamins and minerals that contribute to bone density and support overall health.

3. Fatty Fish:

Fatty fish like salmon, mackerel, and sardines are not only excellent sources of vitamin D but also provide omega-3 fatty acids. Omega-3s have anti-inflammatory properties that may contribute to bone health by reducing inflammation in the body. Including fatty fish in your diet can offer a dual benefit for both bone and cardiovascular health.

4. Nuts and Seeds:

Nuts and seeds are rich in several bone-friendly nutrients, including calcium, magnesium, and phosphorus. Almonds, chia seeds, flaxseeds, and sesame seeds are particularly noteworthy. These nutrient-dense snacks can be incorporated into meals, added to yogurt or salads, or enjoyed as a standalone snack.

5. Lean Proteins:

Proteins are essential for bone health, as they contribute to collagen formation, a key structural component of bones. Incorporate lean protein sources such as poultry, fish, beans, lentils, and tofu into your diet. Balancing protein intake with other essential nutrients ensures a holistic approach to bone health.

6. Fortified Foods:

Incorporating foods fortified with calcium and vitamin D is a strategic way to enhance your nutrient intake. Fortified cereals, plant-based milk, and certain fruit juices can be valuable additions to your diet, especially for individuals who may have dietary restrictions or limited exposure to sunlight, a natural source of vitamin D.

7. Eggs:

Eggs are not only a versatile and affordable source of protein but also contain vitamin D in the yolk. Including eggs in your diet provides a combination of nutrients that contribute to overall bone health.

8. Whole Grains:

Whole grains, such as quinoa, brown rice, and oats, are rich in magnesium and phosphorus. These minerals play a supportive role in bone mineralization. Choosing whole grains over refined grains ensures a higher nutrient content in your diet.

9. Fruits:

Certain fruits contribute to bone health through their vitamin and mineral content. Oranges and other citrus fruits provide vitamin C, which supports collagen formation. Additionally, fruits like bananas and prunes contain potassium, which can help counteract the negative effects of high-sodium diets on bone health.

10. Cruciferous Vegetables:

Vegetables from the cruciferous family, including Brussels sprouts, cabbage, and cauliflower, contain a variety of nutrients beneficial for bone health. These vegetables provide a mix of vitamins, minerals, and antioxidants that support overall well-being.

11. Beans and Legumes:

Beans and legumes are rich in calcium, magnesium, and other essential nutrients for bone health. Incorporate black beans, kidney beans, lentils, and chickpeas into soups, salads, or main dishes to boost your fiber and nutrient intake.

12. Low-Fat Dairy Alternatives:

For individuals who are lactose intolerant or prefer non-dairy options, low-fat or non-fat dairy alternatives such as almond milk, soy milk, or coconut milk can be suitable choices. Ensure that these alternatives are fortified with calcium and vitamin D for optimal bone health benefits.

13. Lean Meats:

Lean meats, such as chicken and turkey, provide a good source of protein and essential nutrients like phosphorus. Including these lean protein options in your diet supports bone health while maintaining a balanced and varied nutritional profile.

14. Seaweed and Sea Vegetables:

Seaweed and sea vegetables, such as nori and wakame, are rich in minerals like calcium, magnesium, and iodine. These nutrient-dense additions can be incorporated into salads, soups, or used as wraps for a unique and flavorful boost to your bone-friendly diet.

15. Cheese:

Cheese is a concentrated source of calcium and protein. While it should be consumed in moderation due to its calorie and fat content, incorporating small amounts of cheese into meals can contribute to overall bone health.

An osteoporosis-friendly diet is a diverse and colorful tapestry of nutrient-rich foods that collectively contribute to bone health. By incorporating a variety of sources of calcium, vitamin D, magnesium, and other essential nutrients, individuals can craft a plate that not only supports bone density but also promotes overall well-being.

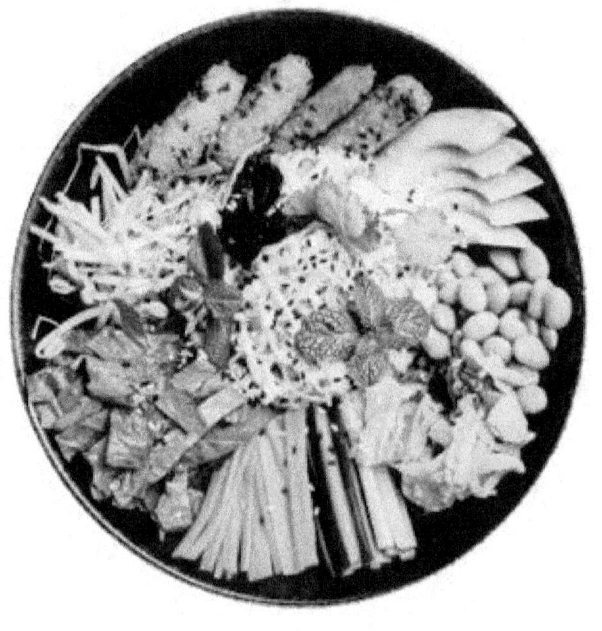

CHAPTER 4

DELICIOUS AND NOURISHING RECIPES

Breakfast Boosts for Bones

1. Green Goddess Smoothie Bowl

Ingredients:

- 1 cup spinach leaves (fresh or frozen)
- 1/2 avocado
- 1/2 banana (frozen)
- 1/2 cup Greek yogurt
- 1/2 cup almond milk (fortified with calcium and vitamin D)
- 1 tablespoon chia seeds
- 1/2 teaspoon honey (optional)
- Toppings: sliced almonds, kiwi, and a sprinkle of flaxseeds

Preparation:

1. In a blender, combine spinach, avocado, banana, Greek yogurt, almond milk, and chia seeds.
2. Blend until smooth and creamy.
3. Pour the smoothie into a bowl.
4. Top with sliced almonds, kiwi slices, and a sprinkle of flaxseeds.
5. Drizzle honey on top if desired.

Portion Size: One serving

Nutritional Information:

- o Calories: 350
- o Protein: 15g
- o Calcium: 400mg
- o Vitamin D: 100IU

2. Salmon and Avocado Toast

Ingredients:

- 2 slices whole-grain bread (fortified with calcium)
- 1/2 avocado
- 100g smoked salmon

- 1 teaspoon lemon juice

- Fresh dill for garnish

- Salt and pepper to taste

Preparation:

1. Toast the whole-grain bread slices.

2. Mash the avocado and spread it evenly on the toasted bread.

3. Top with smoked salmon.

4. Drizzle with lemon juice.

5. Garnish with fresh dill, salt, and pepper.

Portion Size: One serving

Nutritional Information:

- o Calories: 320

- o Protein: 20g

- o Calcium: 150mg

- o Vitamin D: 80IU

3. Yogurt Parfait with Berries and Almonds

Ingredients:

- 1 cup plain Greek yogurt
- 1/2 cup granola (fortified with calcium)
- 1/2 cup mixed berries (blueberries, strawberries, raspberries)
- 2 tablespoons sliced almonds
- 1 teaspoon honey

Preparation:

1. In a glass or bowl, layer Greek yogurt, granola, mixed berries, and sliced almonds.
2. Repeat the layers.
3. Drizzle with honey on top.

Portion Size: One serving

Nutritional Information:

- Calories: 400
- Protein: 20g
- Calcium: 300mg
- Vitamin D: 120IU

4. Spinach and Feta Omelette

Ingredients:

- 2 large eggs
- 1 cup fresh spinach, chopped
- 2 tablespoons feta cheese, crumbled
- 1/4 cup diced tomatoes
- 1 teaspoon olive oil
- Salt and pepper to taste

Preparation:

1. In a bowl, whisk the eggs.
2. In a nonstick pan, warm the olive oil over medium heat.
3. Add chopped spinach and sauté until wilted.
4. Pour the whisked eggs over the spinach.
5. Sprinkle feta cheese and diced tomatoes.
6. Fold the omelette in half after cooking until the edges are firm.
7. Season with salt and pepper.

Portion Size: One serving

Nutritional Information:

- o Calories: 280
- o Protein: 18g
- o Calcium: 150mg
- o Vitamin D: 60IU

5. Chia Seed Pudding with Mango

Ingredients:

- 3 tablespoons chia seeds
- 1 cup almond milk (fortified with calcium and vitamin D)
- 1/2 teaspoon vanilla extract
- 1 tablespoon maple syrup
- 1/2 cup diced mango

Preparation:

1. Combine the almond milk, maple syrup, vanilla extract, and chia seeds in a bowl.
2. Stir well, cover, and refrigerate overnight.
3. Give it a thorough stir in the morning.
4. Top with diced mango before serving.

Portion Size: One serving

Nutritional Information:

- o Calories: 250
- o Protein: 6g
- o Calcium: 300mg
- o Vitamin D: 100IU

6. Whole Grain Pancakes with Berry Compote

Ingredients:

- 1/2 cup whole wheat flour
- 1/2 cup oat flour
- 1 teaspoon baking powder
- 1/2 teaspoon cinnamon
- 1/2 cup almond milk (fortified with calcium and vitamin D)
- 1 egg
- 1 tablespoon honey
- Berry Compote: mixed berries, 1 tablespoon maple syrup

Preparation:

1. In a bowl, mix whole wheat flour, oat flour, baking powder, and cinnamon.
2. In another bowl, whisk together almond milk, egg, and honey.
3. Mix the dry and wet ingredients together until they are well blended.
4. Heat a skillet over medium heat and ladle the batter onto it.
5. Cook on one side until bubbles appear, then turn and continue cooking.
6. For the compote, simmer mixed berries with maple syrup until they release juices.
7. Serve pancakes with berry compote.

Portion Size: Two pancakes with compote

Nutritional Information:

- Calories: 350
- Protein: 10g
- Calcium: 200mg
- Vitamin D: 80IU

7. Quinoa Breakfast Bowl

Ingredients:

- 1/2 cup cooked quinoa
- 1/2 cup plain Greek yogurt
- 1 tablespoon almond butter
- 1/2 banana, sliced
- 1 tablespoon pumpkin seeds
- Drizzle of honey

Preparation:

1. In a bowl, layer cooked quinoa, Greek yogurt, and almond butter.
2. Top with banana slices and pumpkin seeds.
3. Drizzle with honey.

Portion Size: One serving

Nutritional Information:

- Calories: 380
- Protein: 15g
- Calcium: 250mg
- Vitamin D: 70IU

Lunches that Support Bone Strength

1. Salmon and Quinoa Salad

Ingredients:

- 4 oz grilled salmon
- 1/2 cup cooked quinoa
- Mixed salad greens
- Cherry tomatoes, halved
- Cucumber, sliced
- Avocado, diced
- Olive oil and lemon dressing
- Salt and pepper to taste

Preparation:

1. Season the salmon with salt and pepper, grill until cooked.
2. In a bowl, mix cooked quinoa, salad greens, cherry tomatoes, cucumber, and avocado.
3. Top with grilled salmon.
4. Drizzle with olive oil and lemon dressing.

Portion Size: One serving

Nutritional Information:

- o Calories: 450
- o Protein: 25g
- o Calcium: 150mg
- o Vitamin D: 200IU

2. Vegetable and Lentil Soup

Ingredients:

- 1 cup green or brown lentils, cooked
- 1 onion, diced
- 2 carrots, diced
- 2 celery stalks, chopped
- 1 zucchini, diced
- 4 cups vegetable broth
- 1 can diced tomatoes
- 1 teaspoon dried thyme
- Salt and pepper to taste
- Fresh parsley for garnish

Preparation:

1. In a large pot, sauté onion, carrots, celery, and zucchini until softened.
2. Add cooked lentils, vegetable broth, diced tomatoes, thyme, salt, and pepper.
3. Simmer for 20-30 minutes.
4. Garnish with fresh parsley before serving.

Portion Size: One serving

Nutritional Information:

- Calories: 320
- Protein: 18g
- Calcium: 80mg
- Vitamin D: 0IU

3. Chicken and Broccoli Quinoa Bowl

Ingredients:

- 4 oz grilled chicken breast, sliced
- 1/2 cup cooked quinoa
- Broccoli florets, steamed
- Red bell pepper, sliced

- 1 tablespoon olive oil

- Lemon juice

- Garlic powder, salt, and pepper to taste

Preparation:

1. Season chicken breast with garlic powder, salt, and pepper; grill until cooked.
2. In a bowl, combine cooked quinoa, steamed broccoli, and sliced red bell pepper.
3. Top with grilled chicken.
4. Drizzle with olive oil and lemon juice.

Portion Size: One serving

Nutritional Information:

- Calories: 380
- Protein: 30g
- Calcium: 60mg
- Vitamin D: 120IU

4. Spinach and Mushroom Whole Wheat Wrap

Ingredients:

- 1 whole wheat wrap
- 1 cup fresh spinach leaves
- 1/2 cup mushrooms, sliced
- 1/4 cup feta cheese, crumbled
- Hummus
- Salt and pepper to taste

Preparation:

1. In a pan, sauté mushrooms until tender.
2. Warm the whole wheat wrap.
3. Cover the wrap with a layer of hummus.
4. Add fresh spinach, sautéed mushrooms, and crumbled feta.
5. Season with salt and pepper.
6. Wrap and enjoy!

Portion Size: One serving

Nutritional Information:

- o Calories: 320
- o Protein: 15g
- o Calcium: 200mg
- o Vitamin D: 80IU

5. Quinoa Stuffed Bell Peppers

Ingredients:

- 2 bell peppers, halved
- 1 cup cooked quinoa
- 1 can black beans, drained and rinsed
- Corn kernels
- Diced tomatoes
- 1/2 cup shredded cheddar cheese
- Taco seasoning
- Fresh cilantro for garnish

Preparation:

1. Preheat the oven to 375°F (190°C).
2. In a bowl, mix cooked quinoa, black beans, corn, diced tomatoes, and taco seasoning.
3. Stuff bell peppers with the quinoa mixture.

4. Top with shredded cheddar cheese.

5. Bake peppers for 20 to 25 minutes, or until they are soft.

6. Garnish with fresh cilantro.

Portion Size: Two pepper halves

Nutritional Information:

o Calories: 380

o Protein: 20g

o Calcium: 180mg

o Vitamin D: 40IU

6. Mediterranean Chickpea Salad

Ingredients:

- 1 can chickpeas, drained and rinsed

- Cherry tomatoes, halved

- Cucumber, diced

- Red onion, finely chopped

- Kalamata olives, sliced

- Feta cheese, crumbled

- Olive oil and balsamic vinegar dressing

- Fresh oregano for garnish

Preparation:

1. In a bowl, combine chickpeas, cherry tomatoes, cucumber, red onion, olives, and feta cheese.
2. Drizzle with dressing made of balsamic vinegar and olive oil.
3. Toss gently to combine.
4. Garnish with fresh oregano.

Portion Size: One serving

Nutritional Information:

- Calories: 420
- Protein: 18g
- Calcium: 250mg
- Vitamin D: 60IU

7. Turkey and Spinach Wrap

Ingredients:

- 1 whole grain wrap
- 4 oz turkey slices
- 1 cup fresh spinach leaves
- 1/2 avocado, sliced

- Greek yogurt dressing

- Salt and pepper to taste

Preparation:

1. Lay out the whole grain wrap.

2. Layer with turkey slices, fresh spinach, and sliced avocado.

3. Drizzle with Greek yogurt dressing.

4. Season with salt and pepper.

5. Wrap and enjoy!

Portion Size: One serving

Nutritional Information:

- Calories: 350

- Protein: 25g

- Calcium: 120mg

- Vitamin D: 100IU

Dinners for Building Better Bones

1. Baked Salmon with Lemon-Dill Sauce

Ingredients:

- 6 oz salmon fillet
- 1 tablespoon olive oil
- Lemon zest
- Fresh dill, chopped
- Salt and pepper to taste

Preparation:

1. Preheat the oven to 400°F (200°C).
2. Place the salmon on a baking sheet.
3. Drizzle with olive oil and sprinkle lemon zest, fresh dill, salt, and pepper.
4. Bake the salmon for 15 to 20 minutes, or until it is thoroughly done.
5. Serve with additional lemon wedges if desired.

Portion Size: One serving

Nutritional Information:

- o Calories: 350
- o Protein: 25g
- o Calcium: 100mg
- o Vitamin D: 300IU

2. Quinoa and Vegetable Stir-Fry

Ingredients:

- 1/2 cup cooked quinoa
- Mixed vegetables (broccoli, bell peppers, snap peas)
- 4 oz tofu, cubed
- 2 tablespoons soy sauce
- 1 tablespoon sesame oil
- Ginger and garlic, minced

Preparation:

1. In a wok or skillet, sauté ginger and garlic in sesame oil.
2. Add tofu and stir-fry until golden.
3. Add mixed vegetables and cook until tender-crisp.
4. Stir in cooked quinoa and soy sauce.
5. Toss until well combined and heated through.

Portion Size: One serving

Nutritional Information:

- o Calories: 380
- o Protein: 18g
- o Calcium: 120mg
- o Vitamin D: 40IU

3. Chicken and Vegetable Kebabs

Ingredients:

- 6 oz chicken breast, cut into cubes
- Cherry tomatoes
- Zucchini, sliced
- Red onion, cut into chunks
- Olive oil
- Lemon juice
- Rosemary, chopped
- Salt and pepper to taste

Preparation:

1. Preheat the grill or oven.
2. Thread chicken, cherry tomatoes, zucchini, and red onion onto skewers.
3. Drizzle with olive oil, lemon juice, chopped rosemary, salt, and pepper.
4. Cook the chicken thoroughly on a grill or in the oven.
5. Serve with a side of whole-grain rice.

Portion Size: One serving

Nutritional Information:

- Calories: 320
- Protein: 30g
- Calcium: 80mg
- Vitamin D: 120IU

4. Vegetarian Spinach and Chickpea Curry

Ingredients:

- 1 can chickpeas, drained and rinsed
- 2 cups fresh spinach leaves
- 1 onion, diced

- 2 tomatoes, chopped

- 1 cup coconut milk

- Curry powder, turmeric, and cumin

- Garlic and ginger, minced

Preparation:

1. Fry the ginger, garlic, and onion in a skillet until aromatic.

2. Add chickpeas, tomatoes, and spices; cook for 5 minutes.

3. Add the coconut milk and let it boil so the flavors combine.

4. Add fresh spinach and cook until wilted.

5. Serve over brown rice or quinoa.

Portion Size: One serving

Nutritional Information:

- Calories: 400

- Protein: 15g

- Calcium: 120mg

- Vitamin D: 0IU

5. Turkey and Sweet Potato Skillet

Ingredients:

- 6 oz ground turkey
- Sweet potatoes, diced
- 1 bell pepper, chopped
- 1 can black beans, drained and rinsed
- Chili powder, cumin, and paprika
- 1 tablespoon olive oil
- Fresh cilantro for garnish

Preparation:

1. In a skillet, brown ground turkey in olive oil.
2. Add diced sweet potatoes, bell pepper, and spices.
3. Cook until sweet potatoes are tender.
4. Add the black beans and heat through, stirring.
5. Garnish with fresh cilantro before serving.

Portion Size: One serving

Nutritional Information:

- Calories: 380
- Protein: 22g

o   Calcium: 90mg

o   Vitamin D: 40IU

6. Mushroom and Spinach Stuffed Chicken Breast

Ingredients:

- 6 oz chicken breast
- 1 cup mushrooms, chopped
- 2 cups fresh spinach
- 1/4 cup feta cheese, crumbled
- Garlic powder, salt, and pepper
- Olive oil

Preparation:

1. Preheat the oven to 375°F (190°C).
2. Butterfly the chicken breast.
3. Sauté mushrooms and spinach in olive oil until wilted.
4. Add salt, pepper, and garlic powder to the chicken.
5. Fill the chicken with sautéed mushrooms, spinach, and feta.

Bake the chicken for 25 to 30 minutes, or until it is thoroughly done.

Portion Size: One serving

Nutritional Information:

- o Calories: 350
- o Protein: 30g
- o Calcium: 120mg
- o Vitamin D: 80IU

7. Baked Eggplant Parmesan

Ingredients:

- 1 medium-sized eggplant, sliced
- 1 cup whole wheat breadcrumbs
- 2 eggs, beaten
- Tomato sauce
- Mozzarella cheese, shredded
- Parmesan cheese, grated
- Fresh basil for garnish

Preparation:

1. Preheat the oven to 400°F (200°C).

2. Dip eggplant slices in beaten eggs, then coat with breadcrumbs.

3. Place on a baking pan, then bake till golden brown.

4. In a baking dish, layer baked eggplant with tomato sauce and cheeses.

5. Repeat the layers.

6. Bake until cheese is melted and bubbly.

7. Garnish with fresh basil before serving.

Portion Size: One serving

Nutritional Information:

o Calories: 380

o Protein: 20g

o Calcium: 250mg

o Vitamin D: 120IU

Snacks and Treats for Healthy Bones

1. Greek Yogurt and Berry Parfait

Ingredients:

- 1 cup plain Greek yogurt
- Mixed berries (blueberries, strawberries, raspberries)
- 2 tablespoons granola (fortified with calcium)
- 1 teaspoon honey

Preparation:

1. Arrange Greek yogurt, granola, and mixed berries in a glass or bowl.
2. Repeat the layers.
3. Drizzle with honey on top.

Portion Size: One serving

Nutritional Information:

- Calories: 220
- Protein: 15g
- Calcium: 200mg
- Vitamin D: 80IU

2. Almond and Apricot Energy Bites

Ingredients:

- 1 cup almonds
- 1 cup dried apricots
- 1 tablespoon chia seeds
- 1 tablespoon honey
- 1/2 teaspoon vanilla extract
- Pinch of salt
- Shredded coconut for rolling (optional)

Preparation:

1. In a food processor, blend almonds until finely chopped.
2. Add dried apricots, chia seeds, honey, vanilla extract, and a pinch of salt.
3. Blend until the mixture comes together.
4. Roll into bite-sized balls and optionally roll in shredded coconut.

Portion Size: Two energy bites

Nutritional Information:

- o Calories: 180
- o Protein: 5g
- o Calcium: 60mg
- o Vitamin D: 0IU

3. Cucumber and Hummus Stuffed Peppers

Ingredients:

- Mini sweet peppers
- Hummus
- Cucumber, thinly sliced

Preparation:

1. Cut mini sweet peppers in half and remove seeds.
2. Spoon a tablespoon of hummus into each side of a pepper.
3. Top with thinly sliced cucumber.

Portion Size: One serving

Nutritional Information:

- o Calories: 80
- o Protein: 3g
- o Calcium: 20mg
- o Vitamin D: 0IU

4. Dark Chocolate-Dipped Strawberries

Ingredients:

- Fresh strawberries
- Dark chocolate (70% cocoa or higher)
- Chopped nuts (almonds, pistachios) for topping

Preparation:

1. Melt dark chocolate in a heatproof bowl.
2. Dip each strawberry into the melted chocolate.
3. Place on parchment paper and sprinkle with chopped nuts.
4. Allow the chocolate to set before serving.

Portion Size: Five strawberries

Nutritional Information:

- o Calories: 150
- o Protein: 2g
- o Calcium: 40mg
- o Vitamin D: 0IU

5. Cheese and Whole Grain Crackers Platter

Ingredients:

- Assorted cheeses (cheddar, mozzarella, brie)
- Whole grain crackers
- Grapes
- Walnuts

Preparation:

1. Spread a tray with different kinds of cheeses.
2. Add whole grain crackers, grapes, and walnuts.
3. Serve as a delightful and customizable snack.

Portion Size: One serving

Nutritional Information:

- o Calories: 250

- o Protein: 10g

- o Calcium: 200mg

- o Vitamin D: 0IU

6. Banana and Almond Butter Roll-Ups

Ingredients:

- Whole grain tortilla

- 1 banana

- Almond butter

- Cinnamon (optional)

Preparation:

1. Top a whole grain tortilla with almond butter.

2. Place a peeled banana on one end and roll it up.

3. Optionally, sprinkle with cinnamon.

Portion Size: One serving

Nutritional Information:

- o   Calories: 300
- o   Protein: 7g
- o   Calcium: 80mg
- o   Vitamin D: 0IU

7. Frozen Yogurt Berry Bites

Ingredients:

- Greek yogurt
- Mixed berries (blueberries, raspberries)
- Honey

Preparation:

1. Mix Greek yogurt with a drizzle of honey.
2. Spoon yogurt into silicone ice cube molds.
3. Add a few berries to each mold.
4. Freeze until solid and pop out the yogurt bites.

Portion Size: Four yogurt bites

Nutritional Information:

- o   Calories: 120

- o   Protein: 5g

- o   Calcium: 60mg

- o   Vitamin D: 0IU

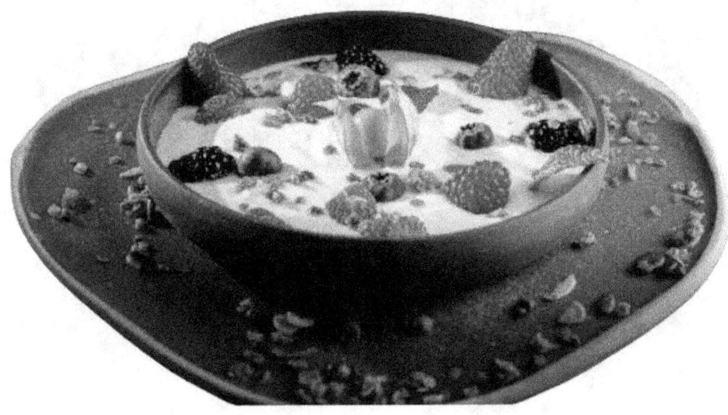

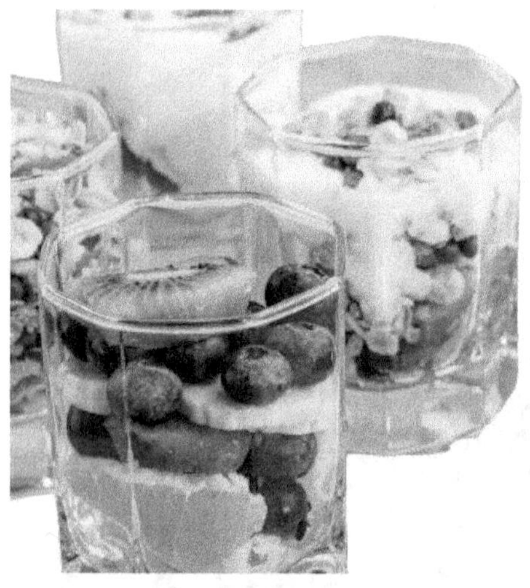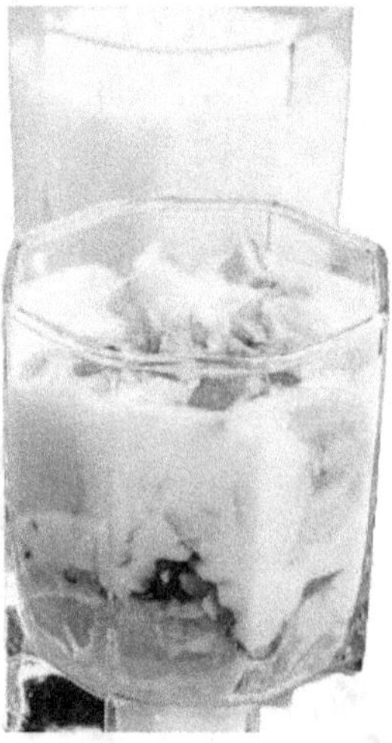

CHAPTER 5

MEAL PLANNING FOR STRONG BONES

30-Day Meal Plan

DAY 1:

Breakfast: Quinoa and Greek Yogurt Parfait

Lunch: Salmon and Quinoa Salad

Dinner: Baked Salmon with Lemon-Dill Sauce

Snack: Greek Yogurt and Berry Parfait

DAY 2:

Breakfast: Almond and Apricot Energy Bites

Lunch: Vegetable and Lentil Soup

Dinner: Quinoa and Vegetable Stir-Fry

Snack: Almond and Apricot Energy Bites

DAY 3:

Breakfast: Banana and Almond Butter Roll-Ups

Lunch: Chicken and Vegetable Kebabs

Dinner: Chicken and Broccoli Quinoa Bowl

Snack: Cucumber and Hummus Stuffed Peppers

DAY 4:

Breakfast: Spinach and Mushroom Whole Wheat Wrap

Lunch: Mushroom and Spinach Stuffed Chicken Breast

Dinner: Vegetarian Spinach and Chickpea Curry

Snack: Dark Chocolate-Dipped Strawberries

DAY 5:

Breakfast: Quinoa Stuffed Bell Peppers

Lunch: Turkey and Spinach Wrap

Dinner: Turkey and Sweet Potato Skillet

Snack: Cheese and Whole Grain Crackers Platter

DAY 6:

Breakfast: Frozen Yogurt Berry Bites

Lunch: Mediterranean Chickpea Salad

Dinner: Baked Eggplant Parmesan

Snack: Greek Yogurt and Berry Parfait

DAY 7:

Breakfast: Breakfast Boost Bowl

Lunch: Quinoa and Vegetable Stir-Fry

Dinner: Quinoa Stuffed Bell Peppers

Snack: Almond and Apricot Energy Bites

DAY 8:

Breakfast: Almond and Apricot Energy Bites

Lunch: Chicken and Vegetable Kebabs

Dinner: Baked Salmon with Lemon-Dill Sauce

Snack: Cucumber and Hummus Stuffed Peppers

DAY 9:

Breakfast: Banana and Almond Butter Roll-Ups

Lunch: Mushroom and Spinach Stuffed Chicken Breast

Dinner: Turkey and Spinach Wrap

Snack: Dark Chocolate-Dipped Strawberries

DAY 10:

Breakfast: Quinoa and Greek Yogurt Parfait

Lunch: Spinach and Mushroom Whole Wheat Wrap

Dinner: Chicken and Broccoli Quinoa Bowl

Snack: Cheese and Whole Grain Crackers Platter

DAY 11:

Breakfast: Quinoa and Greek Yogurt Parfait

Lunch: Salmon and Quinoa Salad

Dinner: Baked Salmon with Lemon-Dill Sauce

Snack: Greek Yogurt and Berry Parfait

DAY 12:

Breakfast: Almond and Apricot Energy Bites

Lunch: Vegetable and Lentil Soup

Dinner: Quinoa and Vegetable Stir-Fry

Snack: Almond and Apricot Energy Bites

DAY 13:

Breakfast: Banana and Almond Butter Roll-Ups

Lunch: Chicken and Vegetable Kebabs

Dinner: Chicken and Broccoli Quinoa Bowl

Snack: Cucumber and Hummus Stuffed Peppers

DAY 14:

Breakfast: Spinach and Mushroom Whole Wheat Wrap

Lunch: Mushroom and Spinach Stuffed Chicken Breast

Dinner: Vegetarian Spinach and Chickpea Curry

Snack: Dark Chocolate-Dipped Strawberries

DAY 15:

Breakfast: Quinoa Stuffed Bell Peppers

Lunch: Turkey and Spinach Wrap

Dinner: Turkey and Sweet Potato Skillet

Snack: Cheese and Whole Grain Crackers Platter

DAY 16:

Breakfast: Frozen Yogurt Berry Bites

Lunch: Mediterranean Chickpea Salad

Dinner: Baked Eggplant Parmesan

Snack: Greek Yogurt and Berry Parfait

DAY 17:

Breakfast: Breakfast Boost Bowl

Lunch: Quinoa and Vegetable Stir-Fry

Dinner: Quinoa Stuffed Bell Peppers

Snack: Almond and Apricot Energy Bites

DAY 18:

Breakfast: Almond and Apricot Energy Bites

Lunch: Chicken and Vegetable Kebabs

Dinner: Baked Salmon with Lemon-Dill Sauce

Snack: Cucumber and Hummus Stuffed Peppers

DAY 19:

Breakfast: Banana and Almond Butter Roll-Ups

Lunch: Mushroom and Spinach Stuffed Chicken Breast

Dinner: Turkey and Spinach Wrap

Snack: Dark Chocolate-Dipped Strawberries

DAY 20:

Breakfast: Quinoa and Greek Yogurt Parfait

Lunch: Spinach and Mushroom Whole Wheat Wrap

Dinner: Chicken and Broccoli Quinoa Bowl

Snack: Cheese and Whole Grain Crackers Platter

DAY 21:

Breakfast: Quinoa and Greek Yogurt Parfait

Lunch: Salmon and Quinoa Salad

Dinner: Baked Salmon with Lemon-Dill Sauce

Snack: Greek Yogurt and Berry Parfait

DAY 22:

Breakfast: Almond and Apricot Energy Bites

Lunch: Vegetable and Lentil Soup

Dinner: Quinoa and Vegetable Stir-Fry

Snack: Almond and Apricot Energy Bites

DAY 23:

Breakfast: Banana and Almond Butter Roll-Ups

Lunch: Chicken and Vegetable Kebabs

Dinner: Chicken and Broccoli Quinoa Bowl

Snack: Cucumber and Hummus Stuffed Peppers

DAY 24:

Breakfast: Spinach and Mushroom Whole Wheat Wrap

Lunch: Mushroom and Spinach Stuffed Chicken Breast

Dinner: Vegetarian Spinach and Chickpea Curry

Snack: Dark Chocolate-Dipped Strawberries

DAY 25:

Breakfast: Quinoa Stuffed Bell Peppers

Lunch: Turkey and Spinach Wrap

Dinner: Turkey and Sweet Potato Skillet

Snack: Cheese and Whole Grain Crackers Platter

DAY 26:

Breakfast: Frozen Yogurt Berry Bites

Lunch: Mediterranean Chickpea Salad

Dinner: Baked Eggplant Parmesan

Snack: Greek Yogurt and Berry Parfait

DAY 27:

Breakfast: Breakfast Boost Bowl

Lunch: Quinoa and Vegetable Stir-Fry

Dinner: Quinoa Stuffed Bell Peppers

Snack: Almond and Apricot Energy Bites

DAY 28:

Breakfast: Almond and Apricot Energy Bites

Lunch: Chicken and Vegetable Kebabs

Dinner: Baked Salmon with Lemon-Dill Sauce

Snack: Cucumber and Hummus Stuffed Peppers

DAY 29:

Breakfast: Banana and Almond Butter Roll-Ups

Lunch: Mushroom and Spinach Stuffed Chicken Breast

Dinner: Turkey and Spinach Wrap

Snack: Dark Chocolate-Dipped Strawberries

DAY 30:

Breakfast: Quinoa and Greek Yogurt Parfait

Lunch: Spinach and Mushroom Whole Wheat Wrap

Dinner: Chicken and Broccoli Quinoa Bowl

Snack: Cheese and Whole Grain Crackers Platter

Quick and Easy Meal Prep Tips

Batch Cooking:

- Prepare larger quantities of recipes, especially those that can be easily reheated or frozen.
- Divide into single-serving portions for quick and convenient meals throughout the week.

Pre-Chopped Ingredients:

- Chop vegetables, fruits, and other ingredients in advance.
- Store them in airtight containers in the refrigerator for easy access during meal prep.

Marinate Proteins:

- Marinate proteins such as chicken, fish, or tofu in advance.
- This enhances flavor and reduces cooking time when it's time to prepare a meal.

Pre-Cook Grains and Quinoa:

- Cook a large batch of quinoa, brown rice, or other grains at the beginning of the week.
- Use them as a base for various meals, saving time on cooking each day.

Create a Salad Bar:

- Wash and chop salad greens and veggies and store them in separate containers.
- Assemble quick salads by combining ingredients from the "salad bar."

Prepare Snack Packs:

- Portion out snacks like Greek yogurt, nuts, or fresh fruit into grab-and-go containers.
- This makes it easy to reach for a healthy snack without additional prep.

Pre-Portioned Smoothie Packs:

- Pre-portion smoothie ingredients into zip-top bags and freeze.

- In the morning, blend with liquid for a quick and nutritious breakfast.

Label and Date:

- Label containers with the name of the dish and the date it was prepared.

- This helps keep track of freshness and ensures you use older meals first.

Invest in Quality Containers:

- Use BPA-free, microwave-safe containers for storing and reheating meals.

- Opt for containers with multiple compartments for keeping components separate.

Plan and Prep on Weekends:

- Dedicate a portion of the weekend to meal planning and prep.
- Cook larger meals that can be portioned for the upcoming week.

Cook Once, Eat Twice:

- Plan meals with leftovers in mind.
- Cook extra portions of proteins or grains to repurpose into different dishes.

Use Slow Cooker or Instant Pot:

- Utilize these appliances for hands-off cooking.
- Set ingredients in the morning, and return to a ready-to-eat meal in the evening.

Keep Staple Ingredients Stocked:

- Ensure your pantry is stocked with essential items like canned beans, canned tomatoes, and whole grains.
- This allows for quick and versatile meal options.

Portion Control:

- Use a kitchen scale or measuring cups to ensure accurate portion sizes.
- This helps in maintaining a balanced and nutrient-dense diet.

Try No-Cook Meals:

- Incorporate meals that require minimal or no cooking, such as salads or wraps.
- This is especially helpful on busy days.

Prep Breakfast the Night Before:

- Overnight oats, chia pudding, or pre-made smoothie packs can streamline breakfast.
- Refrigerate them overnight for a hassle-free morning.

Create a Weekly Menu:

- Plan your meals for the week ahead of time.
- This helps streamline grocery shopping and ensures you have all necessary ingredients.

Multitask in the Kitchen:

- While one component is cooking, work on chopping or preparing another.
- This maximizes efficiency during meal prep.

Rotate Ingredients:

1. Use common ingredients across multiple recipes to reduce the number of different items to prep.
2. For example, if a recipe calls for spinach, plan other meals that also use spinach.

Stay Flexible:

- Be open to adjusting your meal plan based on fresh produce or ingredients on sale.
- Flexibility allows for a more dynamic and cost-effective approach to meal prep.

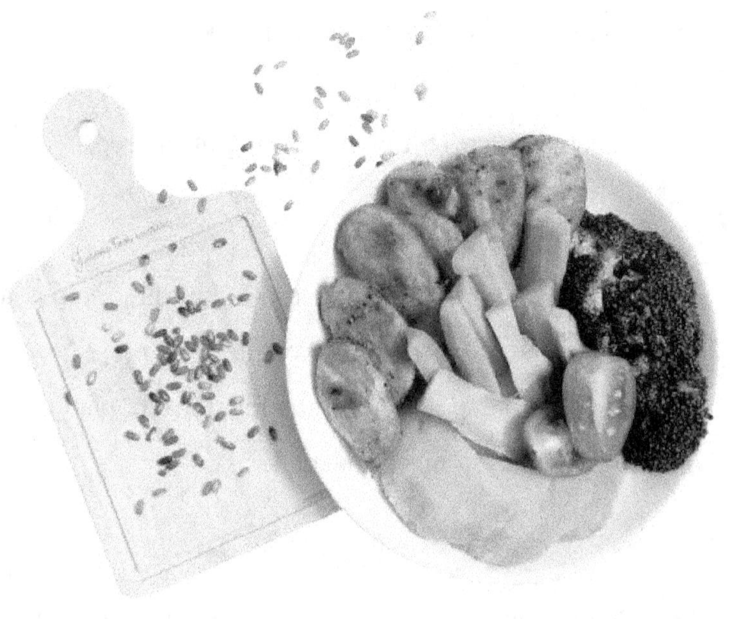

In concluding this journey towards optimal bone health through the OSTEOPOROSIS DIET COOKBOOK FOR WOMEN, we've embarked on a flavorful and nourishing exploration of recipes designed to reverse, cure, and prevent osteoporosis. The path to stronger bones is not just a matter of dietary choices; it's a holistic commitment to wellness that encompasses nutrition, exercise, and a mindful approach to self-care.

Throughout this cookbook, we've delved into the intricacies of osteoporosis, understanding its nuances, risk factors, and preventive measures. We've empowered ourselves with knowledge, recognizing that our choices today lay the foundation for a future of resilient and vibrant bone health.

The importance of nutrition in fortifying our bones has been a central theme, and the diverse array of recipes provided offers a symphony of flavors that not only nourish the body but also delight the taste buds. From the hearty Breakfast Boosts to the nutrient-packed Dinners for Building Better

Bones, each recipe is a step towards a stronger, healthier you.

But this journey extends beyond the kitchen. The inclusion of a 30-Day Meal Plan provides a practical roadmap, making it easier to integrate these bone-boosting recipes into your daily life. Meanwhile, the bonus section on exercises for bone health complements your culinary efforts, creating a well-rounded approach to your overall well-being.

As you savor these recipes, engage in physical activities, and make conscious choices, remember that this is a personal odyssey, one that honors your body and invests in a future of strength and resilience. Small changes today can yield significant dividends tomorrow, and the commitment you've shown to your bone health is a testament to your dedication to a life well-lived.

In the spirit of embracing wholesome living, let this cookbook be your companion on the journey towards fortified bones, a nourished body, and a vibrant life. Here's to your health, your strength, and the endless possibilities that lie ahead. May you savor each meal and each moment, knowing that you are taking positive steps towards a future of vitality and well-being. Cheers to the incredible journey you've embarked upon, one that celebrates the power of nutrition, movement, and self-care in creating a life of lasting wellness.

Thank you for reading this book.

Scan the QR code below to gain more books from this author.

THE BONUS

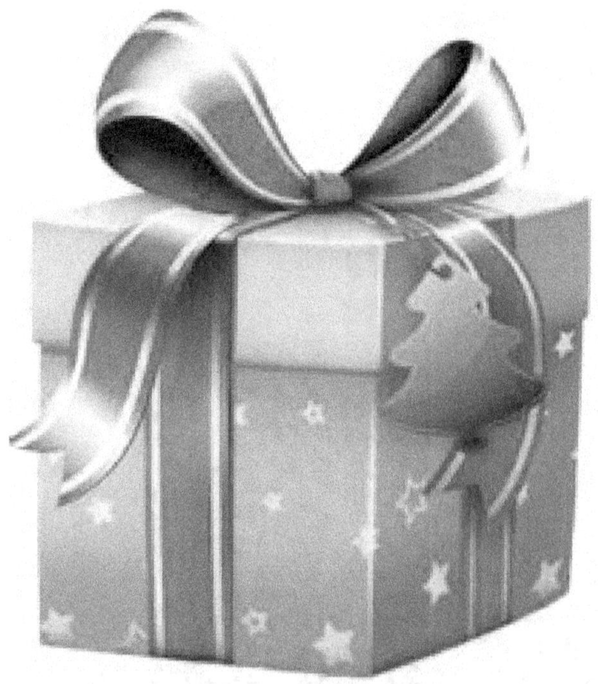

20-Suitable Exercises for Bone Health

Weight-Bearing Aerobic Exercises:

1. Brisk Walking:

- Duration: 30 minutes, 3-4 times a week.
- Tip: Use proper walking shoes and maintain good posture.

2. Jogging or Running (if medically suitable):

- Duration: 20-30 minutes, 2-3 times a week.
- Tip: Choose soft surfaces to reduce impact on joints.

3. Dancing (Low-Impact):

- Duration: 30 minutes, 2-3 times a week.
- Tip: Engage in dance styles with gentle movements.

Strength Training Exercises:

4. Bodyweight Squats:

- Repetitions: 10-15 squats, 2-3 sets.
- Tip: Focus on proper form, keeping knees over ankles.

5. Lunges:

- Repetitions: 10 lunges per leg, 2-3 sets.
- Tip: Take a step forward, keeping the front knee over the ankle.

6. Wall Sits:

- Duration: 30-60 seconds, 2-3 sets.
- Tip: Keep your back against the wall, thighs parallel to the ground.

7. Modified Push-Ups:

- Repetitions: 8-12 push-ups, 2-3 sets.
- Tip: Perform push-ups on your knees to reduce intensity.

8. Resistance Band Exercises:

- Exercises: Bicep curls, lateral raises, leg press.
- Repetitions: 10-15 reps, 2-3 sets for each exercise.

Balance and Stability Exercises:

9. Tai Chi:

- Duration: 30 minutes, 2-3 times a week.
- Tip: Join a Tai Chi class for proper guidance.

10. Yoga:

- Duration: 30-60 minutes, 2-3 times a week.
- Tip: Choose yoga poses that focus on balance and flexibility.

11. Pilates:

- Duration: 30-45 minutes, 2-3 times a week.
- Tip: Include exercises that engage the core and improve posture.

12. Single-Leg Stands:

- Duration: 30 seconds per leg, 2-3 sets.
- Tip: Hold onto a sturdy surface for support if needed.

13. Heel-to-Toe Walk:

- Duration: 20 steps, 2-3 sets.
- Tip: Walk in a straight line, placing the heel of one foot in front of the toes of the other.

Flexibility and Range of Motion Exercises:

14. Neck Tilts and Turns:

- Repetitions: 10 each side, 2-3 sets.
- Tip: Move slowly and avoid any sudden jerking motions.

15. Shoulder Stretches:

- Repetitions: Hold each stretch for 15-30 seconds, 2-3 sets.
- Tip: Gently stretch the shoulders, avoiding excessive force.

16. Arm Circles:

- Repetitions: 10 circles forward, 10 circles backward, 2-3 sets.
- Tip: Perform this exercise with control to avoid strain.

17. Spine Stretches:

- Exercises: Cat-Cow stretch, Child's pose.
- Repetitions: 10 cycles, 2-3 sets for each exercise.

18. Hamstring Stretches:

- Repetitions: Hold each stretch for 15-30 seconds, 2-3 sets.
- Tip: Stretch both legs while sitting or standing.

Functional Exercises:

19. Sit-to-Stand Exercises:

- Repetitions: 10-15, 2-3 sets.
- Tip: Use a sturdy chair for support if needed.

20. Functional Movements Mimicking Daily Activities:

- Examples: Squatting to pick up objects, carrying groceries.
- Tip: Incorporate daily movements into your exercise routine.

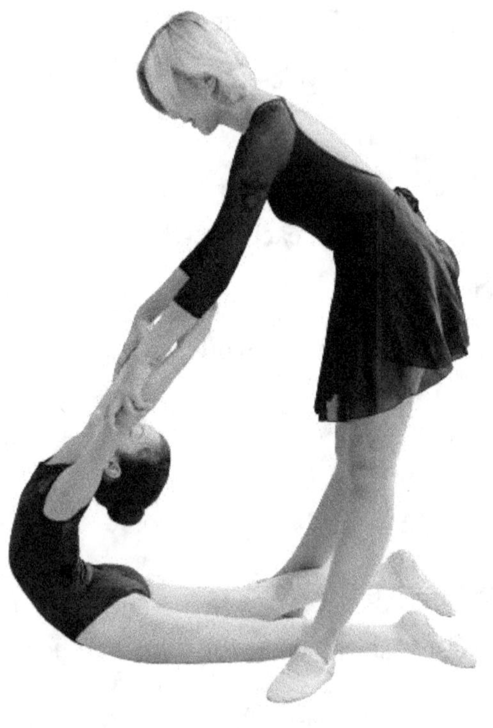

20-Weeks Meal Journal

WEEKLY MEAL JOURNAL

WEEK _______________________   MONTH _______________________

MONDAY

TUESDAY

WEDNESDAY

THURSDAY

FRIDAY

SATURDAY

SUNDAY

SHOPPING LIST

NOTES:

WEEKLY MEAL JOURNAL

WEEK ______________   MONTH ______________

MONDAY

TUESDAY

WEDNESDAY

THURSDAY

FRIDAY

SATURDAY

SUNDAY

SHOPPING LIST

NOTES:

WEEKLY MEAL JOURNAL

WEEK _______________________   MONTH _______________

MONDAY

TUESDAY

WEDNESDAY

THURSDAY

FRIDAY

SATURDAY

SUNDAY

SHOPPING LIST

-
-
-
-
-
-
-
-

NOTES:

-
-
-
-

WEEKLY MEAL JOURNAL

WEEK _______________   MONTH _______________

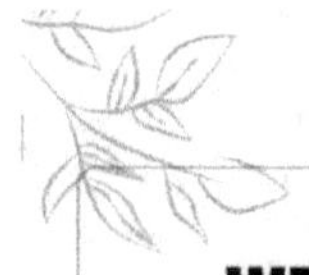

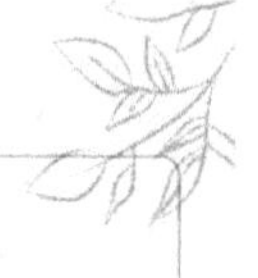

MONDAY

SATURDAY

TUESDAY

SUNDAY

WEDNESDAY

SHOPPING LIST

THURSDAY

FRIDAY

NOTES:

WEEKLY MEAL JOURNAL

WEEK ___________________   MONTH ___________________

MONDAY

SATURDAY

TUESDAY

SUNDAY

WEDNESDAY

SHOPPING LIST

- ○ ___________________
- ○ ___________________
- ○ ___________________
- ○ ___________________
- ○ ___________________
- ○ ___________________
- ○ ___________________
- ○ ___________________

THURSDAY

FRIDAY

NOTES:
- ○ ___________________
- ○ ___________________
- ○ ___________________
- ○ ___________________

WEEKLY MEAL JOURNAL

WEEK ___________________   MONTH ___________________

MONDAY

SATURDAY

TUESDAY

SUNDAY

WEDNESDAY

SHOPPING LIST

- ○ _______________
- ○ _______________
- ○ _______________
- ○ _______________
- ○ _______________
- ○ _______________
- ○ _______________
- ○ _______________

THURSDAY

FRIDAY

NOTES:

- ○ _______________
- ○ _______________
- ○ _______________
- ○ _______________

WEEKLY MEAL JOURNAL

WEEK ______________________   MONTH ______________________

MONDAY

TUESDAY

WEDNESDAY

THURSDAY

FRIDAY

SATURDAY

SUNDAY

SHOPPING LIST

NOTES:

WEEKLY MEAL JOURNAL

WEEK ________________   MONTH ________________

MONDAY

TUESDAY

WEDNESDAY

THURSDAY

FRIDAY

SATURDAY

SUNDAY

SHOPPING LIST

NOTES:

WEEKLY MEAL JOURNAL

WEEK ______________________   MONTH ______________________

MONDAY

SATURDAY

TUESDAY

SUNDAY

WEDNESDAY

SHOPPING LIST

○ ______________________
○ ______________________
○ ______________________
○ ______________________
○ ______________________
○ ______________________
○ ______________________
○ ______________________

THURSDAY

FRIDAY

NOTES:

○ ______________________
○ ______________________
○ ______________________
○ ______________________

WEEKLY MEAL JOURNAL

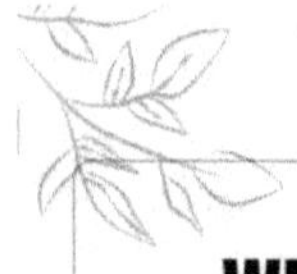
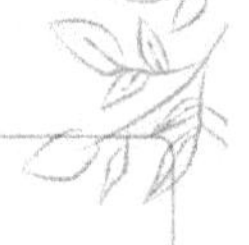

WEEK _______________ MONTH _______________

MONDAY

SATURDAY

TUESDAY

SUNDAY

WEDNESDAY

SHOPPING LIST

- ○ _______________
- ○ _______________
- ○ _______________
- ○ _______________
- ○ _______________
- ○ _______________
- ○ _______________
- ○ _______________

THURSDAY

NOTES:

- ○ _______________
- ○ _______________
- ○ _______________
- ○ _______________

FRIDAY

WEEKLY MEAL JOURNAL

WEEK _______________________   MONTH _______________________

MONDAY

TUESDAY

WEDNESDAY

THURSDAY

FRIDAY

SATURDAY

SUNDAY

SHOPPING LIST

NOTES:

WEEKLY MEAL JOURNAL

WEEK __________________   MONTH __________________

MONDAY

SATURDAY

TUESDAY

SUNDAY

WEDNESDAY

SHOPPING LIST

- ◯ __________________
- ◯ __________________
- ◯ __________________
- ◯ __________________
- ◯ __________________
- ◯ __________________
- ◯ __________________
- ◯ __________________

THURSDAY

FRIDAY

NOTES:

- ◯ __________________
- ◯ __________________
- ◯ __________________
- ◯ __________________

WEEKLY MEAL JOURNAL

WEEK ___________________   MONTH ___________________

MONDAY

TUESDAY

WEDNESDAY

THURSDAY

FRIDAY

SATURDAY

SUNDAY

SHOPPING LIST

- ___________________
- ___________________
- ___________________
- ___________________
- ___________________
- ___________________
- ___________________
- ___________________

NOTES:

- ___________________
- ___________________
- ___________________
- ___________________

WEEKLY MEAL JOURNAL

WEEK ______________________   MONTH ______________________

MONDAY

SATURDAY

TUESDAY

SUNDAY

WEDNESDAY

SHOPPING LIST

THURSDAY

FRIDAY

NOTES:

WEEKLY MEAL JOURNAL

WEEK ___________________   MONTH ___________________

MONDAY

SATURDAY

TUESDAY

SUNDAY

WEDNESDAY

SHOPPING LIST

- ___________________
- ___________________
- ___________________
- ___________________
- ___________________
- ___________________
- ___________________
- ___________________

THURSDAY

FRIDAY

NOTES:

- ___________________
- ___________________
- ___________________
- ___________________

WEEKLY MEAL JOURNAL

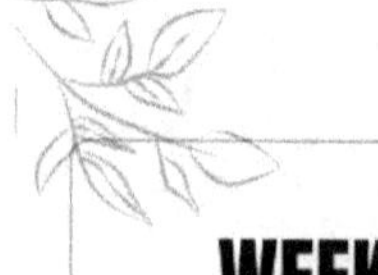
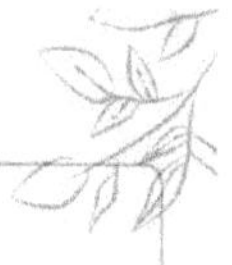

WEEK ___________________ MONTH ___________________

MONDAY

SATURDAY

TUESDAY

SUNDAY

WEDNESDAY

SHOPPING LIST
- ____________________
- ____________________
- ____________________
- ____________________
- ____________________
- ____________________
- ____________________
- ____________________

THURSDAY

FRIDAY

NOTES:
- ____________________
- ____________________
- ____________________
- ____________________

WEEKLY MEAL JOURNAL

WEEK ___________   MONTH ___________

MONDAY

TUESDAY

WEDNESDAY

THURSDAY

FRIDAY

SATURDAY

SUNDAY

SHOPPING LIST

- ○ ___________
- ○ ___________
- ○ ___________
- ○ ___________
- ○ ___________
- ○ ___________
- ○ ___________
- ○ ___________

NOTES:

- ○ ___________
- ○ ___________
- ○ ___________
- ○ ___________

WEEKLY MEAL JOURNAL

WEEK _______________   MONTH _______________

MONDAY

TUESDAY

WEDNESDAY

THURSDAY

FRIDAY

SATURDAY

SUNDAY

SHOPPING LIST

NOTES:

WEEKLY MEAL JOURNAL

WEEK _____________________   MONTH _____________________

MONDAY

TUESDAY

WEDNESDAY

THURSDAY

FRIDAY

SATURDAY

SUNDAY

SHOPPING LIST

- ○ _____________________
- ○ _____________________
- ○ _____________________
- ○ _____________________
- ○ _____________________
- ○ _____________________
- ○ _____________________
- ○ _____________________

NOTES:

- ○ _____________________
- ○ _____________________
- ○ _____________________
- ○ _____________________

WEEKLY MEAL JOURNAL

WEEK —————————— MONTH ——————————

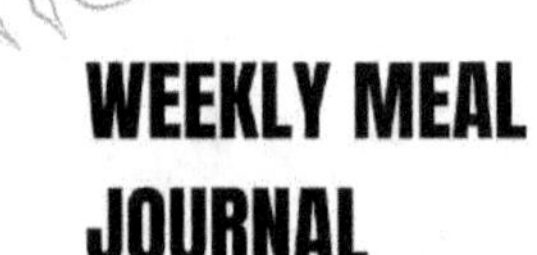

| MONDAY | SATURDAY |

| TUESDAY | SUNDAY |

WEDNESDAY

THURSDAY

SHOPPING LIST

○ ——————————
○ ——————————
○ ——————————
○ ——————————
○ ——————————
○ ——————————
○ ——————————
○ ——————————

FRIDAY

NOTES:

○ ——————————
○ ——————————
○ ——————————
○ ——————————

www.ingramcontent.com/pod-product-compliance
Lightning Source LLC
Chambersburg PA
CBHW070859260726

48661CB00004B/1496